Proven Natural Ways to Lower High Blood Pressure

30 Proven Natural Superfoods To Control & Lower Your High
Blood Pressure

Table of Contents

Chapter 6: Herb Remedies: How Can They Help to Normalize Your Blood Pressure 40

Herbal Remedies for High Blood Pressure 41

Introduction

The rising number of people affected by high blood pressure had brought awareness to the public but being aware of the sickness or its presence is not enough to exclude you from its deadly fang.

For decades, this sickness had been ignored and overlooked because of its silent symptoms which earned it the title of being the "Silent Killer" but as government's efforts are driven towards minimizing if not totally eliminating its presence; attention to this illness is being brought forward to the public.

If you are one of those many people who are not comfortable living with the idea that you could be one of those many who is affected by this illness without actually knowing it, this book, *"Proven Natural Ways to Lower High Blood Pressure: Healthy Lifestyle, Mind Empowerment, and Natural Remedies"* is prepared to equip you with the basic knowledge about high blood pressure and how to reverse it naturally if you have it without the use of drug medications.

Furthermore, while we are into the treatment of high blood pressure, we likewise should be aware of its preventive measures. Know all the important facts about this silent killer and live a healthier life!

Thanks again for downloading this book, I hope you enjoy it and please don't forget to leave us an honest review ☺!

P.S. Before you get started I recommend you joining our e-mail newsletter to receive updates for any upcoming new book releases or promotions. You can sign-up for free and as a bonus you'll also receive our "7 Fitness Mistakes You Don't Know You're Making" training video series. Please visit:

www.helpmeworkout.com/gift/

Chapter 1 – Overview on High Blood Pressure

High blood pressure is one of the primary contributing causes of death in the United States. According to the recent report released by the Center for Disease and Control Prevention, about 75 million American adults have high blood pressure. To give you a quick calculation, that's one out of every three adult Americans or around 29% of the American population. Approximately $46 billion are spent by the nation each year to cover health care services and medications. This also includes missed days of work due to hypertension.

Symptoms of high blood pressure are sometimes so mild that it's hard to detect. However, its results can be deadly and therefore must be taken with utmost concern. Left untreated, high blood pressure, also known as "hypertension can damage and left scars to the arteries which can also be found even in people who are normally calm and relaxed. The "Silent Killer", as it carries no initial symptoms, is a long-term illness which can eventually lead to complications and death.

How Can High Blood Pressure Occur?

High blood pressure is the impact of the blood created against the wall of the arteries as it circulates inside the human body. The blood pressure is determined by the amount of blood pumped by the heart against its resistance as it flows through the arteries.

When there are some blockades like cholesterol build up, scarring or plaque in the arteries, it affects the elasticity of the arterial walls and narrows the way of the blood stream, thereby creating more pressure as the heart pumps harder to get the blood through just so it can reach the different parts of the body.

Such increase in pressure can damage the muscles and valves in the heart and may result in heart failure. Damages to the vessels supplying blood and oxygen to kidneys and brain eventually create a negative impact on these body organs.

Too much pressure in the blood vessels and arterial walls can cause serious problems. Generally, healthy arteries are made of semi-flexible tissues and muscles that are fine, smooth, elastic and stretchable so blood flows easily through them when the heart starts to pump mildly. However, when there are blockades, the heart is forced to pump more thereby stretching the walls of the arteries and if done too much, it could break the lining of the arterial walling. Once blood vessels are broken, it could lead to stroke, kidneys malfunction, peripheral vascular failure or heart attack which causes death to the majority of its victims.

It is, therefore, essential to keep your blood pressure at a level to reduce the risk of blood vessels from getting overstretch beyond the limit and injured. Uncontrolled blood pressure increases the risk of more serious health or medical problems to occur.

Chapter 2: The Danger of Having High Blood Pressure

High blood pressure is steadily increasing in modern societies due to an unhealthy lifestyle. This can be very disturbing if you are not fully aware of its implications in your health condition, but if you do, you can look for effective options to reverse its effects.

High blood pressure can silently do some serious to your body system long before the onset of symptoms. Taking it for granted can result to a disability, a life of suffering, and even a serious heart attack. People who are left untreated of high blood pressure die of ischemic heart disease or poor blood flow. Others die of stroke.
A shift in lifestyle and treatment can help control your high blood pressure to reduce these life-threatening risks. Now, let's take a look to some of the damages it can cause to your body.

Damage to your Arteries

When your arteries are healthy, they are flexible, elastic, and strong with a smooth inner lining along the walls to let the blood flows freely as it circulates around the body. This is a vital process as it supplies nutrients and oxygen to vital tissues and organs. When the bloodstream is clogged, it causes an increase in pressure in the arterial wall as the heart pumps vigorously to let the blood flows in. As a result, you will be experiencing the following:

Damaged and Narrowed Arteries

When you have an unhealthy lifestyle, your body can collect fats from your diet and stored them in your arteries, clogging the flow of the bloodstream and your artery walls become less elastic. This limits the flow of blood in your body.

Aneurysm

Eventually, the constant pressure of blood against the weakened artery lining may cause a part of the wall to form a bulge. This condition is called "an aneurysm". An aneurysm can rupture anytime and cause an internal bleeding in any artery but mostly it occurs in the aorta or the largest artery in your body.

Damage to the Heart

Since your heart pumps blood to your body, uncontrolled high blood pressure can do damage to your heart in a number of ways.

Coronary Artery Disease

This condition affects the arteries that supply blood to the body. The disease narrows down the arteries and limits the blood to flow freely through the arteries. When you have this illness, you can experience irregular heart rhythms known as (arrhythmias), chest pains or irregular heart attack.

Enlarged Left Heart

When your heart is forced to exert vigorously in order to pump blood into your body, it causes the left ventricle to become stiffen or thickens (left ventricular hypertrophy). These changes also limit the ventricle's ability to pump blood thereby increasing the risk of a heart failure, heart, attack and sudden cardiac death.

Heart Failure

Eventually, strain on your heart caused by the high blood pressure weakens your heart muscles and make them work less efficiently. If this continues to go on, this condition will simply wear out your heart will wear out in time and fail and if there's some damage caused by heart attack, they add more to the existing problem.

Damage to the Brain

Like your heart, the brain depends on the supply of blood to nourish it so it can work properly to survive. However, when there is high blood pressure, it can cause problems including what we have here below.

Transient Ischemic Attack (TIA)

Considered as a "mini stroke", this condition is a temporary disruption of the blood supply to your brain. Transient Ischemic Condition is often caused by atherosclerosis or a blood clot. Both of these can arise when there is high blood pressure and the presence of the TIA is a warning that you're at risk for a full-blown stroke.

Stroke

When part of your brain is deprived of oxygen and nutrients supplied through your blood vessels, it will cause the death of your brain cells. So, when you have high blood pressure that it left uncontrolled or neglected, this can cause the narrowing, rupture or leaks in your blood vessels leading to the brain.

High blood pressure can likewise cause blood clotting in the arteries blocking the blood flow to your brain and causing a stroke.

Dementia

This condition is associated with problems in cognitive abilities – thinking, speaking, reasoning, memory, vision, and movements. There are various causes of dementia including vascular dementia which is attained through narrowing and blockage of the arteries that supply blood to the brain. It can also be resulted by a stroke that causes an interruption in the blood flow leading to the brain. In any of these cases, it's the high blood pressure that mainly causes it.

Mild Cognitive Impairment

There is a transition stage, which occurs between the changes in understanding, and memory as one grows old and the more serious problems developed when one got an Alzheimer's disease. Like dementia, this results from blocked blood flow when arteries are damaged by high blood pressure.

Damage to your kidneys

Normally, it's the function of your kidneys to filter excess waste and fluids from your blood, though this process depends on your healthy blood vessels. When high blood pressure injures your blood vessels leading to your kidneys, it may cause numerous types of kidney diseases (nephropathy). If you have diabetes, this can even worsen the damage.

Kidney Failure

Generally, kidney failure is caused by high blood pressure as it brings damage both to the large arteries leading to your kidneys and the tiny blood vessels (glomeruli) within the kidneys. Damage to either of these two affects the normal function of your kidneys hindering it from effectively filtering waste from the blood. In the end, a dangerous level of waste and fluids can accumulate in your body and may ultimately require dialysis or a kidney transplant.

Kidney Scarring

Glomerulosclerosis is a type of kidney damage caused by scarring of the glomeruli (glue-MER-u-li). The glomeruli are tiny clusters of blood vessels within your kidneys that filter fluid and waste from your blood. Glomerulosclerosis can leave your kidneys unable to filter waste effectively, leading to kidney failure.

Kidney Artery Aneurysm

This is a type of an aneurysm leading to the kidney. One potential cause of this disease is atherosclerosis which damages and weakens the artery wall. In the long run, a weakened artery can cause a section to form an aneurysm which can rupture anytime and cause a life-threatening bleeding internally.

Chapter 3: Causes and Symptoms

It's not easy to identify the exact cause of high blood pressure, but numerous factors and conditions that may somehow have contributed to its development. Here are among them.

- Obesity or overweight
- Lack of Physical Activity
- Too much consumption of salt and alcohol
- Smoking
- Genes and family history including high blood pressure
- Unmanageable stress
- Chronic Kidney Ailments
- Thyroid and Adrenal Disorders
- Sleep Apnea

Essential Hypertension

In the United States, more than 95% of reported high blood pressure cases, the underlying cause is not determined. For this type of high blood pressure, people in the medical world call it as the "essential hypertension".

Mysterious as it is, essential hypertension has been somehow linked to certain risk factors. High blood pressure tends to affect more males than their female counterparts and is likewise observed to run in the family.

Added to these, age and race also play a vital role. Blacks living in the United States are twice likely to have high blood pressure compared to Whites but the gap decreases at around age 44. Many black women have the highest reported incidence of high blood pressure at the age of 65 and above.

Other factors that affect essential hypertension are diet and lifestyle. The link between salt and high blood pressure had long been established. Japanese people living in the northern islands of Japan are known to consume more salt per capita than people in the rest of the world and they've got the highest incidence of essential hypertension. Conversationally, who don't use salt to their food have no traces of essential hypertension.

People with high blood pressure are hypersensitive that even a small excess of salt added to what is normally needed by the body can send their blood pressure to soar up. Other factors that count in the presence of essential high blood pressure are an insufficiency in calcium, magnesium, and potassium, chronic alcohol consumption, obesity, and diabetes.

Secondary Hypertension

Contrary to essential high blood pressure is the Secondary High Blood Pressure or "secondary hypertension". With this type of high blood pressure, the direct cause is somehow pinpointed and kidney disease ranks the highest among the many causes of secondary hypertension.

This type of high blood pressure can be triggered by tumors and other abnormalities which cause the adrenal glands to produce excess amounts of hormones that elevate the blood pressure.   Those that can send blood pressure to rise up include:

- Pregnancy
- Birth control pills particularly those that include estrogen
- Drugs that constrict blood vessels

Chapter 4: Preventive Measures for High Blood Pressures

Making an extra effort to prevent the onset of high blood pressure can help in the reduction of stroke, heart attack, and many other serious illnesses that can lead to death. If you are at risk for high blood pressure, it's best for you to take these preventive measures.

Preventive Factors You Can Control

Some factors like, age and genes including family medical histories are something beyond your control. Therefore, if you want to prevent the onset of high blood pressure, you need to focus on the risk factors that you can change. We are not able to do something about our age or what constitute our DNA but we can always change our lifestyle for a better and healthy one. Here are some ways to consider in shifting to a healthy lifestyle.

Maintain a Normal and Healthy Weight

Maintaining a healthy weight is crucial when it comes to hypertension. Overweight and obesity can lead to more complications which can eventually lead to death. People who are overweight need to lose weight and if you are normally-weight, then avoid adding more pounds. Finally, if you are carrying extra weight, lose as much as ten pounds to help prevent the occurrence of high blood pressure. There are online resources to help you know your ideal weight and your body mass index (BMI).

Eat a Balanced Diet

Eating a healthy balanced diet can help keep your blood pressure under control. Eat foods that are rich in potassium while keeping a limit on calories, fat, sodium, and sugar. DASH Diet is known to help in managing high blood pressure.

Cut Back Sodium Consumption

The higher the sodium intake you have, the higher the blood pressure rises. Therefore, it is better to cut down on your sodium intake by avoiding foods that are high in sodium content like packaged foods and processed food. It may also help to avoid adding salt to your meals.

Limit Alcohol Intake

Drinking too much alcohol thickens the blood and therefore create more pressure for the heart to have it flowed smoothly and freely. Therefore, avoid having more than a drink in a day.

Have a Regular Exercise

It takes the activity to make one healthy and physical activity is crucial when referring to high blood pressure. The more exercise you have to your body, the better. However, even a little bit of exercise can do so much to lessen the risk of hypertension. Start doing a moderate exercise for about 30 minutes. If you can do this three times a day, the better it can be for you to start with.

Monitor Your Blood Pressure

After you have done with the ways stated above, make sure that you regularly monitor your blood pressure. To do this, you can either go to a clinic or do this at home. Since hypertension often shows no apparent symptoms, only the blood pressure reading can give you a definite measurement of your blood pressure. Blood pressure reading in the range of 120-139/80-89 millimeters of mercury (mmHg) puts you at an increased risk of developing high blood pressure.

Finally, take a look at your lifestyle and see what among your habits need to be transformed. Try conquering small goals like eating fruits and vegetables instead of junk foods in between meals. Make these habits as part of your daily routine.

Chapter 5: Proven Ways to Control High Blood Pressure Without Medication

Although we have introduced here some preventive measures to get away from having high blood pressure, still we know it's not really that easy to make a 360 degrees shift in your lifestyle. With the kind of modern life we have today when almost everyone is constantly on the go, we fill in our stomachs with instant food right out of the package. We know that these foods are far from being healthy and unless you're determined to change your ways, you need to refrain from eating this kind of foods.

What about if you already have that sickness in you?
As I have stated, high blood pressure is a sickness that need not be ignored. Deaths related to high blood pressure run to almost 100,000 each year and is still rapidly increasing. Some people simply ignore their problem while others choose medications with negative effects. But, nowadays, majority resort back to the use of simple natural remedies to treat high blood pressure. There are many natural remedies proven over the years to combat high blood pressure.

Before considering drug medication for your hypertension problem, take note of the following facts.

- ✓ Pharmaceutical companies are considered as one of the most lucrative business in the 21st Century.

- ✓ The number of hospitals has grown exponentially these past decades. Before it was believed to be due to baby boomers or those in their retirement age, however, recent studies are showing that people tend to rely more on doctors nowadays for every aspect of their physical health.

- ✓ Insurance rates and coverage have grown too high partly due to inflated medical and prescriptions cost.

Though drugs are definitely not bad for they also have their own purpose in life and are likewise beneficial to our society, still there are drugs that are harmful is some ways as they are harsh and carry deadly side-effects in many ways.

Nonetheless, millions of people are still choosing to forego using medications with dangerous side effects and instead resort to the holistic and natural treatment of high blood pressure. With holistic treatment, we refer to the kind of treatment that views the wholeness of a person. That is, instead of focusing on the treatment of a disease, the holistic approach looks at an individual's overall physical, emotional, mental, and spiritual wellbeing before recommending treatment.

This holistic approach to natural treatment might involve a nutritional diet, regular exercise, meditation, and much more. Attacking high blood pressure on many different angles can completely cure the person without the use of drug medication!

How Can One Benefit From the Natural Treatment

Beside from the avoidance of the life-threatening side effects of drugs, there are various reasons why you need to consider treating high blood pressure naturally. Here are some things you need to consider in doing so.

Weight Loss

People who undergone natural treatments learn not only how they are cured of their high blood pressure, but also managed to shed extra pounds. When you know the right kind of food to eat, you will minimize your cravings and therefore can lose 1-2 pounds in a week.

Improved Stamina and Energy

Because of proper nutrition, you will experience improved stamina and energy and therefore can do things that you can enjoy. When one has a healthy body, life can be better for him that with those who doesn't have a healthy and fit body.

Reviving Youthfulness

When you have high blood pressure, you are missing out on major vitamins and minerals that are needed by the body. Vitamins and minerals like calcium, magnesium, and zinc play a vital role in normalizing your blood pressure. When you have adequate of these substances, then you will feel much younger and alive.

Controlling Hypertension

There are over a thousand listed benefits for exercising and controlling your blood pressure is one of them. Learn a simple exercise which you can do every day for 20-30 minutes and you will eventually experience that your blood pressure is going back to normal.

No Side Effects!!!

Unlike medicine drugs, the only side effect you can get from taking natural remedy is feeling bad about not trying it sooner.

Natural Ways to Control High Blood Pressure Without Medication

Changing lifestyle is said to show a normalized blood pressure in around 86 percent of those who have high blood pressure. Therefore, if you want to reverse your hypertension, you need to normalize your weight. Once you begin to have healthier eating habits, then you can begin to adapt to the following strategies to beat your hypertension.

Step #1 – Walk, walk, walk!

Start to walk as much as you can. Work up to walk slowly for longer and longer distances. Try power walking – brisk walking for about 30 minutes in a day. This activity can increase your oxygen supply in the body to keep your heart function smoothly and efficiently. As you get used to power walking, try to increase your speed and distance while you increase strength and stamina.

Step #2 – Inhale, Exhale!

Take time to breathe deeply. Sit in a chair with your back straight. Breathe as deeply as you can for five or ten minutes. Stress hormones elevate a kidney enzyme called renin which actually raises blood pressure. By slowly deep breathing and expanding your belly, you exhale all the tension out of your body. Adding qi gong, tai chi or yoga to that deep breathing is another great stress buster.

Step #3 – Take More Potassium, Reduce Sodium in Your Diet

Watch out for the amount of animal protein in your diet because eating too much of it causes a rise in your body acid levels and actually diminishes your potassium level. Therefore, it is better to add more naturally potassium-rich foods to your meals such as fresh fruits and vegetables, whole grain, dairy and poultry products, meat, and fish.

Highly potassium-rich foods include broccoli, halibut, tuna, spinach, parsley, oranges, bananas, avocados, strawberries, crimini mushrooms, Brussels sprouts, kidney beans, tuna, eggplant, apricots, dried prunes, raisins, cantaloupe, honeydew melon, potatoes, peas, squash, chard, sweet potatoes, bell peppers, cucumbers, tomatoes, and cabbage.

Buy as little processed food and limit your sodium intake by buying food that contains a higher level of sodium. You can avoid this by reading food labels as you will become more aware of the amount of salt in every pack of food that you buy in the grocery or supermarket.

People with high blood pressure are sometimes salt-sensitive. Because there are no available test to show if you are sensitive to salt or not, it is, therefore, important to be aware of how much salt you are taking so to be able to reduce as much as possible.

Step #4 – Add Cocoa to Your Diet

A half an ounce of dark chocolate added to your diet contains at least 70 percent cocoa. Dark chocolates contain a substance called "flavanols" which make blood vessel more elastic. The elasticity of blood vessels helps to lower down high blood pressure.

Cocoa flavonols are bioactive derived from cacao beans. Earlier studies on cacao beans disclosed that flavanols can improve cardiovascular functions while lessening the burden on the heart that comes along with aging and heart's stiffening. The study further reveals that the intake of cocoa flavanols reduces the risk of developing cardiovascular diseases.

Step #5 – Alcoholic Beverage Helps, Too!

Having about ¼ -1/2 drink of alcoholic beverage helps to lower your blood pressure. Studies revealed that a small amount of alcohol drink in a day lowers risk of heart disease and protects the heart. However, more than that is sure to be detrimental.

Step #6 – Avoid Caffeine

Studies about caffeine show that it causes high blood pressure by tightening blood vessels. This highlights the effects of stress and raises high blood pressure as well. Therefore, you can avoid a blood pressure spike when you are stressed by using decaf coffee and other drinks.

Drinking hibiscus coffee is associated with a significant decrease in hypertension. A study has proven that drinking 3 cups of hibiscus coffee a day for a period of over 6 weeks brought a significant change in the level of blood pressure of participants. The Journal of Nutrition had published that hibiscus tea can cause the blood pressure to lower down naturally and was likewise effective in adults who are classified as either mildly hypertensive or pre-hypertensive.

Step #7 – Avoid Working Too Much!

Working for more than 41 hours in a week can add hypertension to the list of health risks since people who works too much tend to eat less healthy food and do not have enough time to exercise. Overload of responsibilities and tasks adds stress to your daily routine which could later bring you more health issues. Try to have a rest and relaxation as often as you can.

More Alternative Treatments to Include in Your Diet!

There are many other ways to normalize your high blood pressure and you can include these in your diet. Here are some of them.

Selenium

Selenium, copper, and zinc are just some of the compound elements that can be helpful. There are studies that show how people with heart diseases are often deficient of these elements. You can have supplements of these elements by taking multivitamins in your diet. Sources of selenium are meat, walnuts, Brazil nuts, dark greens, and wheat. Zinc is usually found in beans, meat, and dairy while copper is present in seafood, legumes, nuts, and dark, leafy vegetables.

Beta Glucan

This substance lowers cholesterol level and likewise lowers blood pressure resulting from high cholesterol. You can get beta-glucan from oat bran and maitake mushroom. This substance further aids in moving waste materials out of the human body. A 200 milligram of oat bran (about a teaspoon) to be taken daily can lower hypertension.

L_Argine

By taking 2 grams of L-Arginine a day can reduce systolic pressure by 20 points after you have taken the supplement for 2 days. It is largely due to the amino acid that helps the body to produce nitric acid which regulates blood pressure and cholesterol.

Fish Oil or Flaxseed

Known as Omega 3 Fatty Acid, Fish oil is beneficial for those who are suffering from hypertension for fish oil protects the heart as well as lowers the blood pressure. For vegetarians, you may try flaxseed. Consuming just a tablespoon of the flax seed daily can help you lower down your hypertension by nine points.

Chapter 6: Herb Remedies: How Can They Help to Normalize Your Blood Pressure

One of the naturally accepted treatments for high blood pressure is the use of herbal as home remedies. The recent increase in the level of shifting from drug medication is largely due to the fact that there could be a rapid increase in the statistics for hypertension sufferer or the fact that people are fed up with the side effects resulting from the use of drug medication, not to say the costly prescriptions.

Herbal Remedies for High Blood Pressure

Arjuna (Terminalia Arjuna)

This amazing Arjuna plant is associated with high blood pressure treatment. Its bark is known for its remarkable remedy of the sickness by protecting the heart and stopping the bleeding as well as toughening the muscles in the organ while improving the blood circulation.

Triterpene Glycosides and *Coenzymes Q10*, compound substances that help the heart and the arterial blood vessels to function properly are said to be abundant in Arjuna plant. Regular use of this herbal medicine will help eliminate the risk of hypertension and prevent further damage to the heart and the rest of vital organs that are affected by high blood pressure.

Dandelion (Taraxacum Officinale)

If you have an issue on fluid retention, dandelion can be useful as it helps increase the urine flow and helps lower blood pressure. One can benefit from the use of dandelions through the elimination of potassium loss which pharmaceutical diuretics often have. However, make sure that when you use these dandelion leaves, they are not treated with pesticides.

Cayenne (Capsicum Annum)

Cayenne aids in thinning the blood, thus lowering the blood pressure. Just use the hot Mexican or Thai seeds like those used in Serranos or African Bird Peppers which are among the hottest of the cayenne products.
To use cayenne for remedy, just take a cup of lukewarm water mixed with one teaspoon of cayenne pepper. Drink the solution for maintenance.

Ginger (Zingiber officinale)

Another herb that is popularly used as a cooking spice is ginger. Though we often consume this home kitchen ingredient, yet most are not aware of its health benefits, including regulating high blood pressure. Ginger is very useful in improving blood flow, treating nausea, relaxing muscles of the arteries, facilitating easy digestion, and easing morning sickness.

Garlic may come in various forms including dry roots, capsules, fresh roots, oils, liquid extracts, powders, supplements, etc. You can eat garlic raw or add it to your delectable dishes.

While ginger is generally proclaimed as safe and effective for hypertension, some people may experience some possible side effects which you must be cautious of – Allergic reactions, gastric disturbance, heartburn problems or mouth irritation.

Guggul (Commiphora Wightii)

Primarily, this herb grows in India but can also be found in other countries in Central Asia and Northern Africa. Studies indicate that this amazing herb has the capability to reduce bad cholesterol LDL and likewise address health issues related to psoriasis, arteriosclerotic vascular disease, and cardiac ischemia.

Garlic (Allium Sativum)

For a long time, we have recognized garlic as an aromatic ingredient we used for food seasoning. However, we failed to realize that garlic actually lowers down our blood pressure by ten percent. Even when it's in the form of gel capsules, garlic still has the same effect.

Garlic also possesses the capability to lessen blood clotting and clears your arteries of bad cholesterols and plaques. For better performance, daily consumption of 1 or 2 cloves for 90 days is enough to prevent and minimize the effects of high blood pressure. It can either be eaten raw or included in your meals.

Reishi (Ganoderma lucid)

This is one species of mushroom associated with lowering of blood pressure. The mushroom is almost inedible but available in capsule form.

Hawthorn (Crataegus app)

Hawthorn causes arterial walls to relax and dilate and it can take many weeks or months to show any effect.

Hawthorn (Crataegus Laevigata)

Hawthorn is beneficial in widening arterial blood vessels, preventing the growth of atherosclerosis, decreasing cholesterol levels, enhancing blood circulation, and regulating heartbeat.

You can consume this herb by drinking it in tea form using its dried leaves and flowers. You may also include hawthorn berry supplements in your dietary plan. Whatever form you use, you can experience a 2.60 HG reduction in your blood pressure level. All these results established hawthorn as a highly trusted herbal treatment for blood pressure.

Celery (Apium Graveolens)

Celery had been used as a remedy since the early age and it occupies a unique among herbal remedies for blood pressure. It aids in increasing the flow of urine and Indians is used to use it in their daily life having recognized celery as one of the best remedies for high blood pressure.

Cocoa (Theobroma Cacao)

Another amazing herb that is associated with lowering high blood pressure effectively is the Cocoa. It works as antioxidants like tea and red wine. According to researchers, a daily dose of 3.5 ounces of cocoa is effective as taking a daily dose of high blood pressure medication.

Valerian (Valeriana Officinalis)

Valerian relaxes the smooth muscles lining the arterial walls by preventing them from constricting.

Broccoli (Brassica Oleracea var. Italica) and Dark Leafy Greens

Broccoli and dark leafy vegetables are high in vitamins and minerals that are essentially needed by people with high blood pressure. Magnesium and calcium are found in abundance in broccoli and other dark leafy vegetables.

Turmeric (Lucuma Longa)

Turmeric is basically used as a spice used in curries. It has anti-inflammatory and antioxidant properties which lower cholesterol level and strengthen body vessels as well as lowering pressure.

Gingko Biloba

Gingko Biloba is known Chinese herbal remedy for hypertension that improves circulation of the blood and dilates arteries. It likewise improves memory and makes one mentally alert.

Olive Leaf Extract

The extract derived from the olive leaf is used as a remedy for high blood pressure to combat irregular heart beat or what is called as "arrhythmia".

Jaundice Berry

With this herbal remedy, blood flow is facilitated to run smoothly in the arteries by dilating blood vessels through the release of tension on the arteries.

Cayenne

Cayenne is known as the best herb for high blood pressure next to garlic. To get the best results, choose the hottest of the cayenne species. Cayenne is known to result in proper control of blood pressure.

Red Clover

People with high blood pressure tends to have their blood thickened resulting to the extra effort of the heart in pumping blood through the vessels. The pressure therefore against the arteries is heightened causing hypertension. Red clover is best for thinning blood hence, lowering blood pressure, and improving blood circulation. To be used effectively, the red clover needs to be in good state – blossoms must remain purple in color. Brown colored clover is dry and has lost their effectiveness.

Alfalfa

Alfalfa helps in softening hardened arteries while reducing high blood pressure. It plays a vital role in hypertension treatment.

Parsley

Parsley is best in maintaining blood circulation and the whole circulatory system of the body while it lowers high blood pressure.

Gooseberry

Known as "Amla" in India, Gooseberry can be consumed with honey in its juice form. Take 1-2 tablespoon daily on an empty stomach as is a primarily beneficial to people with high blood pressure.

Onion and Honey

A mixture of onion juice and honey can do wonders for people with high blood pressure. Drinking two teaspoons a day of this mixture can reverse the effect of high blood pressure and helps you return to a normal life.

Fenugreek Seed (Trigonella Foenum-Graecum)

Seeds from this plant are known to carry various health benefits including the following:

Lowers Blood Cholesterol

Studies had proven that fenugreek helps in lowering down cholesterol level, particularly that of LDL or low-density lipoprotein. The herb is known to be enriched with steroidal saponins which are associated with the absorption of cholesterol and triglycerides.

Reduces Risks of Heart Disease

Fenugreek leaves contain a high amount of potassium which counters the negative effect of sodium in the body to help control heart beat rate and blood pressure.

Keeps You in Shape

When you include fenugreek in your diet by chewing soaked seeds in the morning on an empty stomach, the natural fiber in the fenugreek can fill up and causes your stomach to swell, suppressing your appetite. This aids you in attaining your weight loss goals as you also tend to lose your cravings for foods.

All the above conditions are beneficial and somehow related to regulating high blood pressure.

Chapter 7: Stress Management: Empowering Mind and Body

It's still debatable whether long-term blood pressure and stress are connected. However, taking measures in order to manage and reduce your stress greatly benefits your overall health including your blood pressure.

The Connection Between Stress and Long-term High Blood Pressure

While experts cannot define the direct relationship between these two, it's quite proven that stressful events can definitely cause temporary increase blood pressure. What you can do in order to avoid long-term high blood pressure is to take preventive measures that will generally benefit your health in both mind and body.

Exercising is a drug-free way of helping you lower your blood pressure and letting you observe healthy lifestyle. It reduces your stress levels as it releases endorphins which are essential in making you feel good about yourself and the things around you. For instance, you can exercise 3-5 times a week for about half an hour in order to reduce your stress level. Other physical activities such as doing household chores, gardening, dancing, swimming, or jogging can also increase your breathing and heart rates, generating benefits in rendering your blood pressure under control.

Remember that under stressful situations, your body produces a rush of hormones which can cause your heart to beat faster for a while and narrowing your blood vessels in the process. There's no strong proof that stress directly results in long-term blood pressure but behaviors such as overeating, smoking, substance abuse and observing poor sleeping habits can all contribute to high blood pressure. Over time, these series of temporary sharp increase of blood pressure can put you into the danger of having a long-term high blood pressure.

On the other hand, stress-related health conditions such as isolation, anxiety, and depression which can be connected to heart disease may not be connected to high blood pressure at all. The reason may be because of the hormones that are produced during the stressful moments.

These hormones can then damage the arteries, exposing you to the risks of heart disease. Additionally, if you are stressed or depressed, you also have the tendency to neglect yourself. This includes the probability of not taking necessary medications that can control your high blood pressure and/or heart condition.

Activities that Can Reduce Blood Pressure

Stress management is a must-observe skill can help you in a lot of ways. Mastering it can help you a healthy lifestyle that can benefit your overall health—both mind and boy—including the regulation of your blood pressure. The following steps may help you get started in how to handle your stress:

Make Your Schedule Simple

One of the most difficult things most of us experience is how to simplify our schedule. Usually, we tend to procrastinate only to find ourselves in a rush to finish our work, projects, assignments, etc. With this hustle and bustle, it's quite normal that our body accepts this as stress which isn't good for our body when accumulated over time.

Eliminate or curtail unnecessary activities that take up a lot of your time. For example, chatting with your friends in Facebook take a great deal of your morning schedule. Instead of doing this, you can choose a more time-worthy schedule wherein you can move around your body or exercise your mind.

Be Conscious of Your Breathing

Breathing is essential for us; after all, we breathe in order to live. When we breathe, each cell in our body takes in the supply of oxygen that contributes to the production of energy in our system. It also allows us to get rid of the toxins our body must eliminate in order to stay healthy.

Unfortunately, most of us take breathing for granted. Busy schedule and fast-paced lifestyle contribute more to our neglect in taking deep breaths which are very important in our health.

You can do simple breathing exercises by doing deep inhalation and exhalation all throughout the day. Take a few deep breaths and let your body relax, letting go of the stressors being accumulated in our body. This process allows you to intake oxygen and actually feed the cells of your body the much-needed supply necessary for your survival.

Do Regular Work Out

In this modern age wherein computers and various gadgets dominate our lifestyle, we tend to be sedentary. Remember that physical activity is a natural stress reliever. With the advice of your doctor, you can plan your exercises starting from simple activities such as walking or jogging. You can also try these various activities:

- Doing household chores and gardening
- Climbing the stairs
- Walking (in the park or any relaxing place)
- Dancing
- Playing tennis, basketball, or dodgeball

Meditate

Meditation has been proven to benefit the health of both our mind and body. It helps us to relax and have that inner calm that is essential to achieving balance.

Back in 2008, Massachusetts General Hospital doctor Randy Zusman asked his patients with high blood pressure to undertake a three-month long meditation-base relaxation program. These patients regularly took medication in order to control their high blood pressure. After the course of three months, 40 out of 60 patients displayed a remarkable drop in their blood pressure levels.

As a result, they were able to lessen their medication intake. The scientific explanation about this is that as the body and mind enter the state of relaxation, nitric oxide can then be formed resulting in the opening of blood vessels, regulating the flow of blood pressure.

Yoga helps you to control your blood pressure. In doing regular stretches, your muscles can become flexible resulting in controlled blood pressure without the use of medications. Stretching exercises develops a series of physiological reactions that may inhibit the stiffening of arteries due to aging.

Develop Good Sleeping Habits

When you are deprived of sleep, you usually gain weight due to the lowering of your *leptin* (the hormone in charge of prompting your brain that you already had enough food eaten) hormone levels and increasing of the biochemical called *ghrelin* which intensifies your appetite to eat.
This bodily reaction greatly affects your eating behavior, making you intake high amounts of calories which your body doesn't need.

Additionally, sleep deprivation also makes your body release higher levels of insulin after you eat, boosting fat storage and exposing you to greater risk of having type-2 diabetes.

Sleep plays an important role in repairing and healing your blood vessels as well as your heart. Lack of it promotes high blood pressure, stroke and heart disease.

According to one study of Harvard Medical School, patients with high blood pressure may experience the hike of their blood pressure levels all throughout the next day upon staying late the night before. In order to help yourself fight off sleep deprivation, here are the best steps that you should observe:

- Consume caffeine only in mornings.
- Set aside your mobile devices and other gadgets after dinner.
- Observe a consistent waking up schedule.
- Avoid using sedatives like Valium, Nyquil, Ambien or even alcohol.
- Take a 15-minute nap every afternoon instead of drinking coffee.

Be Optimistic

Having a positive mindset and attitude greatly helps in promoting your overall health. When you're mind is relaxed, your body automatically creates balance and harmony leading to good health—and regulating your blood pressure levels is one of the benefits of having this inner calm. Quite a number of studies also show that being optimistic tend to give a person a quality and long life. For instance, a happy and contented person who enjoys laughing in the company of his loved ones tends to lead a long life compared to those who suffer depression or have a negative outlook on life.

According to some studies, there is an association between the positive outlook and lower blood pressure. Individuals who have a positive mindset tend to have controlled blood pressure levels; whereas, those who look towards life in a negative perspective have the highest risk of developing high blood pressure. Moreover, positive individuals have the lower percentage of exposing themselves into evolving into cardiovascular disease.

Therefore, if you want to enjoy a quality life until your old age, it's time to recreate your mindset. You can always start in little things. For example, you can marvel at the little things nature gives us like the sunlight, warmth, the sky or even the moon during the night.

Be conscious of your inner voice and how you talk to yourself. Avoid talking about your mistakes or highlighting your worries. Before you are tempted to do that, give yourself some space and assess the situation. While you can see unfavorable aspects, you always have the choice to shed on that matter. Don't forget to laugh in every chance you have. A good one can help lessen your mental burden, even making it easier for you to handle challenging problems.

Chapter 8: How Meditation Can Help in Lowering High Blood Pressure

In addition to the conventional methods of combating high blood pressure, Mindfulness-Based Reduction Technique (MBRS) is gaining followers and practitioners all over the world. By incorporating mindfulness meditation into your lifestyle along with physical fitness activity and weight management, your goal of reducing high blood pressure is achieved and thereby reverse its effect on your body.

According to a research study, to curb blood pressure and ward off hypertension, it is extremely important to keep your mind away from stress and anxiety.

Researchers from Case Western University School of Medicine conducted a study on hundred of patients with hypertension aging 30-60 years old. The program consisted of 8 sessions covering 2 ½ hours each. Participants were then asked to meditate using the body scan exercise for 45 minutes in six days per week. The study resulted in a significant outcome with the result indicating a 1.9-mm Hg decrease in diastolic blood pressure (DBP) and 4.8-mm Hg decrease in systolic blood pressure (SBP). The findings were published in the Psychosomatic Medicine Journal.

In a recent study on blood pressure, distress and coping, it was revealed that through a selected mind-body intervention, a decrease in blood pressure was detected relative to increased coping and decreased psychological distress in young adults conducive to high blood pressure.

Based on these studies, it was proven that meditation can be effective in lowering the level of blood pressure while combating the ill effects of stress and anxiety in the human body.

As you resolve to shift to a healthier lifestyle choice, you must incorporate meditation into your everyday routine. Making a habit of practicing daily or doing meditation exercises even for just 20 minutes is sure to make a big difference on how your body moves, how your mind thinks, and how your body feels.

When your mind and emotions are calm and controllable, you're in a better position to face all the challenges in your life and the goals that you have set for yourself – which in this case happens to be regulating your blood pressure to a normal level.

Those negative feelings including worry, anxiety, and fear plus the regular occurrence of stress as you are constantly exposed to various stressors can be greatly relieved by a daily practice of meditation. As your mind is cleared of muddled thoughts, keeping you stuck in unhealthy behaviors, you will be surprised to see how you would see life in a different viewpoint. All the changes in your life always begin in your mind.

Your mind always has the power over your body – from the tip of your hair down to the tip of your toes. Being able to control your mind and tame it so you can lead it to where you want is an effective way of calming your overall sense so as not to send your heart beating or pumping as it normally does. When you are able to do this, then you are getting rid of the stressors that tend to send your blood pressure up.

Rather than doing the same routine using the same mindset and results that are disappointing, meditation allows you to set the stages for some major shift in your life and this includes, primarily your health.

Managing your Health, Saving Your Life!

Just as human illness is relatively stress-related, meditation works well to relieve you from stress. It likewise helps in treating illnesses. Not only mediation resolve the issue on high blood pressure or hypertension risks but it is also associated with the relief of the following illnesses:

- Skin disorders

- Mild depression

- Pre-menstrual syndrome and dysmenorrhea

- Sleeping apnea and fatigue

- Recurring pain including headaches

- Respiratory issues like asthma and emphysema

- Rheumatoid Arthritis (RA) symptoms

- Gastrointestinal distress

- Irritable bowel syndrome

Health and medical condition like the ones we have here will certainly deprive you of the vitality and live a life of fun and enjoyment. When you let stress weight you down as you are burdened with anxiety and negative thoughts and emotions, it stresses that is in control and not you!

Could there be more satisfying that having a cure against a stress-related illness that is natural? This is what meditation is offering you – A life of happiness – free from the claw of this deadly sickness.

A Way To Do Your Meditation Exercise

To start, find a comfortable place to do your exercise. Though old-timers can do it anywhere and would find it easy to achieve their meditation goal anywhere and anytime, beginners can get easily distracted, hence, you need a more quiet and serene place to meditate. You can either sit on a chair or on the floor as long as you feel comfortable and relaxed. If you need something to soothe your senses, prepare some music.

Start by closing your eyes or just focus your attention on something like maybe the floor near where you are sitting. Then start breathing in and out gently, trying to feel the air as it passes through your nostrils and runs through every part of your body before you slowly take it out through your mouth, Feel every moment – either you focus on your breathing or you focus on the object of your attention.

If you are closing your eyes, imagine of something – an image, an object, a mantra or anything you want to connect with. If you find your mind wandering out of focus, slowly get it back without judging yourself. The goal here is to be able to control your thinking to focus on something and not get affected emotionally but just silently look at it at the present moment.

Focusing on your breathing gives you a new awareness of your life and while you are doing this activity, you may be able to grasp a new meaning to your existence. This could be a simple and quite exercise that could last for a few minutes but out of it, something new – an insight maybe will be revealed to you in a spur of a moment.

Short as it is, you could not imagine the benefits this meditation exercise can bring you – physically, mentally, emotionally, and spiritually. It is for this reason that more and more people resort back to transcendental or mindfulness meditation as a way of treating stress to reverse the effects of high blood pressure or minimize the risks of more serious health problems.

Ideally, set aside 15-30 minutes a day for meditation so calm down your senses and prepare them for facing the daily struggles and challenges in life. This way, your body won't feel threatened and set itself to a fight or flight mode which causes it to produce some hormonal change in your body, sending your heart to produce more pressure and forcing the arterial wall to break.

There are some online resources and tools like the Insight CD System, which you can set up by yourself and so a quick mediation session for 20 minutes or more depending on your preference.

While listening to the CD, you can literally teach your brain to work n synchronization –that is, training your left and right side of the brain to work in consonance in order to create a wide distribution of electrical activity and energy patterns throughout your brain instead of having it confined to limited areas. This tool is designed in agreement with the result of a study which indicates that this full brain synchronization is active at times of intense creativity, clarity, and inspiration.

To sum this up, whether you are doing meditation without the use of the Insight audio CD or any tool like this, make sure that that you incorporate the meditation exercise in your daily activities. Make this a habit, not only to regulate your high blood pressure but a part of a healthy lifestyle. It's a simple step but its lasting result can have a profound and lasting effect on your overall physical health and mental wellbeing.

Conclusion

A great number of hypertension sufferers are now getting tired of experiencing the debilitating effects of drug prescriptions and medication that most opted to resort back to the natural remedies. Now that many are asking if the natural way of treating high blood pressure really works, proven studies answer this question with a big "YES!"

However, natural treatment is a holistic approach that needs to be consolidated into your lifestyle to be able to benefit from it fully. It does not answer to only one area of your life but needs to make a thorough overhauling of your wellbeing.

Now that you have become aware of the extent that natural remedies can do to your goal of bringing down to the normal level your high blood pressure, you can use this knowledge to regulate your blood pressure and manage your hypertension to prevent the onset of other complications or more serious illnesses.

High blood pressure can be a silent killer only if you neglect to give enough attention to your lifestyle. It's not high blood that kills, but it's your failure to create a healthy lifestyle that can give you a better, safer, and longer life!

The next step is to join our e-mail newsletter to receive updates for any upcoming new book releases or promotions. You can sign-up for free and as a bonus you'll also receive our "7 Fitness Mistakes You Don't Know You're Making" training video series. Please visit http://www.helpmeworkout.com/gift/

Finally, if you enjoyed this book, then I'd like to ask you for a favor, would you be kind enough to leave a review for this book on Amazon? It'd be greatly appreciated!

Click here to leave a review for this book on Amazon!

Thank you and good luck!

About the Author

My name is George, I'm a personal trainer from Montreal, Canada. I'll start off by saying I'm not the biggest guy or the most ripped person you'll ever meet and this has never really been my goal. In fact, I started working out to overcome my biggest insecurity when I was younger, which was my self-confidence. This was due to my height measuring only 5 foot 5 inches (168cm), it pushed me down to attempt anything I ever wanted to achieve in life. You may be going through some challenges right now or you may simply want to get more fit and I can certainly relate.

For me personally, I was always interested in the fitness world and wanted to gain some muscle due to the numerous bulling in my teenage years about my height and my overweight body. I figured I can't do anything about my height but I sure can do something about how my body looks like. This was the beginning of my transformation journey. I had no idea where to start but I just got started. I felt lost and scared at times. I was worried that other people would make fun of me for doing the exercises the wrong way. I always wished I had a friend that was next to me who was knowledgeable enough to help me get started and "show me the ropes".

After a lot of work, studying and many many trial and errors, many began to notice how I was getting more fit and how I was beginning to form a strong interest in topic. This led many friends and new faces to come to me and ask me for fitness advice. At first it seemed odd when people asked me to help them get in shape. But what kept me going is when they started to see changes in their own body and told me it's the first time that they actually saw real results! From there, more people kept coming to me and it made me realize after so much reading and studying in this field that it actually did help me but it also allowed me to help others. This is when I decided to go deeper into the fitness world. I'm am now a fully certified personal trainer and I'm also currently doing a bachelors of Kinesiology in University.

All this to say, I started just like you. I've asked myself how I could do it. I've read for countless hours, studied, doubted myself, failed, succeeded, and learned a lot on how our body works. If you are in the position I was once in and you want guidance, don't hesitate and ask... I'll be there to help you out.
Your friend and coach,
George Workout

George Workout

Certified Personal Trainer &
Co-founder, HelpMeWorkout.com

P.S. To keep in touch, please don't forget to <u>sign up to my e-mail newsletter</u>. You can sign-up for free and as a bonus you'll also receive our "7 Fitness Mistakes You Don't Know You're Making" training video series. Please visit: <u>www.helpmeworkout.com/gift/</u>

47013212R00039

Made in the USA
Middletown, DE
14 August 2017